An Illustrated Pocketbook of Hypertension

An Illustrated Pocketbook of Hypertension

Peter F. Semple
*Department of Medicine and Therapeutics,
University of Glasgow, Glasgow, UK*

The Parthenon Publishing Group
International Publishers in Medicine, Science & Technology

A CRC PRES S COMPANY

BOCA RATON   LONDON   NEW YORK   WASHINGTON, D.C.

Published in the USA by
The Parthenon Publishing Group
345 Park Avenue South, 10th Floor
New York, NY 10010, USA

Published in the UK and Europe by
The Parthenon Publishing Group Limited
23–25 Blades Court
Deodar Road
London SW15 2NU, UK

Library of Congress Cataloging-in-Publication Data
Data available on application

British Library Cataloguing in Publication Data

Semple, Peter
   An illustrated pocketbook of hypertension
   1. Hypertension
   I. Title
   616.1'32

ISBN 1-84214-057-4

Copyright © 2003 The Parthenon Publishing Group

Composition by The Parthenon Publishing Group
Printed and bound by T. G. Hostench S.A., Spain

Contents

Introduction

The detection and control of hypertension are the key to preventing stroke, but the goal of attaining normal blood pressure without side-effects is still not consistently achieved.

Overwhelming evidence supports the concept that blood pressure in the population is a continuously distributed variable, bearing a graded relationship to risk of vascular events, so that any definition of hypertension is, by necessity, arbitrary. The line dividing 'normal' from 'high' blood pressures is often set at 140/90 mmHg, although definitions vary. By most criteria, approximately 10–20% of adults will develop raised levels of blood pressure by the time they are middle-aged.

High blood pressure is most strongly predictive of increased risk of stroke, and the increased risk associated with high pressures is almost completely reversed by effective antihypertensive drug therapy. The relationship between blood pressure and risk of coronary events is not as close as for stroke, but there is again evidence that treatment of blood pressure reduces the risk appreciably.

High blood pressure recordings at initial screening tend to fall somewhat if repeated over weeks or months. This is thought to be a reflection of both an attenuation of the alarm reaction and a statistical phenomenon known as regression to the mean. As a method of diagnosis, monitoring of office or clinic blood pressures over relatively long periods of time is increasingly tending to be replaced by either ambulatory measurements taken over 24 hours or home monitoring of blood pressure using validated semi-automatic devices.

Inherited factors are important in the pathogenesis of the most common form of high blood pressure, namely primary or essential hypertension. The specific genes associated with the condition have not yet been identified but some promising lines have been identified.

Interactions between different genes may also be significant. Other factors, such as obesity, insulin resistance, dietary sodium intake, stress and excessive alcohol intake, interact with the genetic substrate.

Only around 5% or less of all hypertensive patients have a recognizable cause of their hypertension. In such cases of so-called secondary hypertension, the hypertension is most often due to underlying renal or renovascular disease, but other, less common causes include syndromes of corticosteroid excess such as primary aldosteronism, and pheochromocytoma and coarctation of the aorta.

Severe hypertension may develop into an accelerated or malignant form but, in developed countries, the incidence has declined steeply in recent years. The clinical diagnosis of malignant hypertension is relatively easy in the presence of bilateral flame-shaped retinal hemorrhages. Such fundal changes are accompanied by fibrinoid necrosis in the arterioles of the kidney, and these are typical of the condition. Moderately raised blood pressure does not usually give rise to symptoms unless a cardiovascular event such as stroke or myocardial infarction has occurred.

High blood pressure has long been recognized as a factor that accelerates the development of atherosclerosis and causes coronary artery disease. In such cases, blood pressure then interacts positively with other factors such as blood levels of cholesterol, cigarette smoking, and obesity.

Because treatment trials in hypertension have shown a somewhat disappointing impact on myocardial infarction compared with stroke and heart failure, there has been a tendency towards an integrated approach to correct risk factors in the individual patient. Various tables have been devised to attempt to quantify individual risk and to facilitate identification of the patients most likely to benefit from drug treatment for high concentrations of blood cholesterol.

Target organs

Brain

The risk of stroke is directly related to arterial pressure, and this graded relationship appears to be maintained even within the normal range of diastolic blood pressure. Meta-analysis of nine prospective observational studies confirmed that there is no convincing evidence of a 'threshold' level of diastolic blood pressure at which risk begins. In general, with sustained increases in diastolic blood pressure of 5, 7.5 and 10 mmHg, there are corresponding increases in stroke risk of 34, 46 and 56%, respectively. Of the factors that predict stroke, blood pressure is dominant, although other independent risk factors have been identified and these include smoking, obesity and plasma levels of fibrinogen.

The incidence of stroke remains particularly low in some less-developed countries where the average diastolic blood pressure may be only 60 mmHg. In China, Japan and parts of Africa, high blood pressure and stroke are common but coronary artery disease is relatively infrequent. This discrepancy, at least in the Far East, is probably due to differences in prevailing levels of blood cholesterol and low-density lipoproteins (LDL).

Just over 10% of all clinical strokes are caused by cerebral hemorrhage. Hemorrhages in hypertension are caused by rupture of microaneurysms that develop on the short penetrating branches of the main cerebral arteries. Such small aneurysms have been identified on arteries 50–220 μm in diameter, principally at sites of branching, and are particularly frequently seen in the distribution of the lateral lenticulo-striate artery. The density of lesions tends to be highest in the putamen, globus pallidus, caudate nucleus, thalamus, external capsule and basis pontis. Hemorrhage into the putamen is especially frequent (Figure 1), and presents as weakness of the contralateral face, arm and

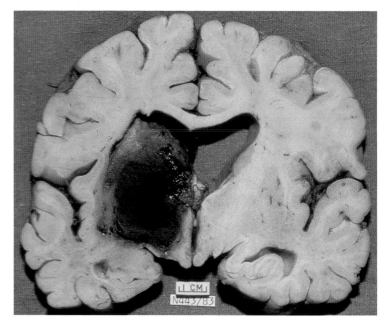

Figure 1 Coronal section of brain showing hemorrhage in the putamen of a patient with hypertension. Bleeding originates from 'miliary' aneurysms in short perforating arteries, as proposed by Charcot and Bouchard in 1889

leg, sometimes with hyperreflexia at an early stage. Large lesions cause hemisensory loss and hemianopia with conjugate deviation of the eyes, reduced consciousness and aphasia, or visuospatial neglect (Figure 2).

Another brain lesion associated with uncontrolled hypertension is a small infarct which evolves into a slit-like space or lacune 0.5–15.0 mm in diameter (Figure 3). These small deep infarcts are often undetectable on computed tomography (CT), and are the result of occlusion of one of the same perforating arteries that rupture in hypertensive cerebral hemorrhage. The arteries immediately proximal to small infarcts show segmental disorganization of the vessel wall, possibly resulting from mechanical disruption of the intima and insudation of plasma constituents. Such changes are seen in small arteries that are close to high-pressure arteries, but not in vessels of the same

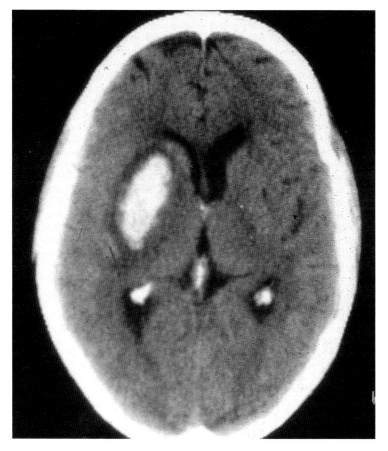

Figure 2 Computed tomography (CT) shows hemorrhage into the right putamen in a patient with uncontrolled hypertension. There was severe hemiplegia and hemianesthesia with visuospatial neglect

caliber at more remote sites. The relative underdevelopment of the muscle and elastic tissue layers of these particular small brain arteries may contribute to their vulnerability. Intraluminal pressures may also be higher in these arteries than in those of similar diameter elsewhere because of their shorter lengths.

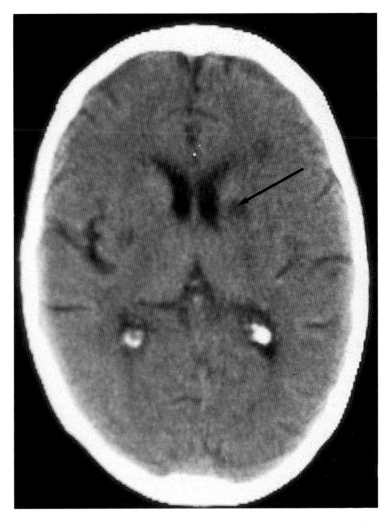

Figure 3 CT showing lacunar infarction at the genu of the internal capsule (arrow) in a patient with poorly controlled hypertension. Infarcts of this type are the result of occlusion of penetrating end arteries. Pure motor hemiparesis is a typical lacunar syndrome

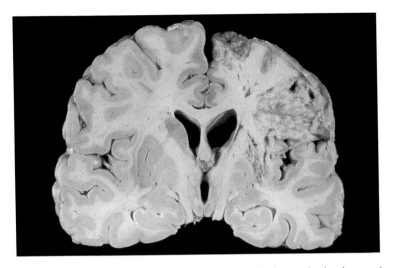

Figure 4 Coronal section of brain showing an established infarct in the distribution of the middle cerebral artery. Infarction in this territory is often the result of occlusion in the extracranial internal carotid artery

Lacunar infarcts resulting from small-vessel disease probably account for up to 20% of ischemic strokes in the developed countries and most usually present as episodes of pure motor hemiparesis, pure sensory stroke or ataxic hemiparesis. Symptoms may evolve progressively over a period of 24–48 hours. Because subcortical white matter is involved, there are no signs of cortical dysfunction such as dysphagia, neglect, agnosia, or apraxia. Transient ischemic attacks may also occur. It is not difficult to understand that the incidences of hemorrhage and lacunar infarction are greatly reduced by effective treatment of chronic hypertension.

Most strokes in Western populations are due to atheromatous disease, often affecting extracranial vessels, especially the origin of the internal carotid artery. This predilection to atheroma is probably explained by the turbulent blood flow at a point of arterial bifurcation causing alterations in endothelial function. Atheroma within the proximal internal carotid artery most often causes cerebral infarction in the

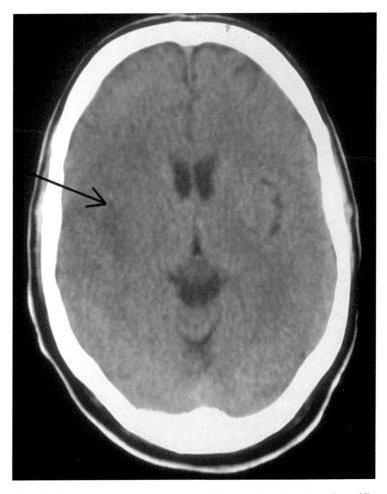

Figure 5 CT showing subtle early changes of infarction (arrow) in the right middle cerebral artery (MCA) territory caused by thrombosis of the internal carotid artery. There is loss of the insular 'ribbon' and slightly reduced attenuation in the superficial MCA territory

distribution of the middle cerebral artery. Vascular occlusion is initiated by rupture of the fibrous cap of an atherosclerotic plaque with superimposed thrombosis. Artery-to-artery embolism is the predominant mechanism of transient ischemic attacks (TIAs) in carotid artery stenosis. In some cases, the fragmented emboli can sometimes be visualized as refractile cholesterol-rich deposits at points where the retinal arterioles branch.

The velocity of blood flow in narrowed vessels is increased, and this acceleration may be detected by Doppler ultrasonography in combination with a two-dimensional image of the structures referred to as the duplex method with color flow imaging. Because Doppler misclassifies a proportion of carotid artery lesions, computed tomographic angiography or magnetic resonance angiography is increasingly used to supplement or replace ultrasonography. Most TIAs in the territory of a stenosed internal carotid artery are caused by either athero-embolism with resultant hemiparesis or amaurosis fugax.

Clinical trials have clearly shown that drug treatment of hypertension reduces the incidence of stroke by about 40% and benefit accrues after relatively short periods of reduction in blood pressure. Benefits are especially seen in men or women of African-American origin and in elderly patients with isolated systolic hypertension or diabetes. Monotherapy is not effective in about 40% of patients; these patients require more than one drug and sometimes several different drugs. Treatment trials have not differentiated between hemorrhagic stroke, lacunar events and large artery disease and cardioembolism. In primary prevention, there is some evidence from the Hypertension Optimal Treatment (HOT) study that aspirin in patients with well-controlled arterial pressures reduces the risk of myocardial events but, if pressures are poorly controlled, then there is little evidence that aspirin is of benefit. In secondary prevention of stroke, results of the PROGRESS trial showed that treatment based on an angiotensin converting enzyme (ACE) inhibitor and thiazide diuretics were effective in reducing risk of re-occurrence of major vascular events, but treatment was not started until at least 2 weeks from the acute event. Benefits extended to patients with normal levels of blood pressure.

There have been concerns about antihypertensive therapy immediately after stroke when cerebral autoregulation is impaired, but there is, as yet, little evidence from clinical trials about the safety (or otherwise) of early antihypertensive therapy. Antiplatelet agents such as aspirin or clopidogrel are also routinely used for prevention of ischemic strokes, and the combination of aspirin and dipyridamole may also be effective. In the presence of large artery atherosclerosis causing carotid or extracranial vertebral artery stenosis, antihypertensive drugs have the potential to cause ischemic events if the degree of narrowing is critical. In practice, such events seem to occur rather infrequently. Symptomatic carotid stenoses greater than 70% are treated by endarterectomy and trials of angioplasty and stent insertion are ongoing. There is less certainty about the role of surgery in asymptomatic patients and various algorithms have been proposed to quantify risk in individual patients.

Retina

Accelerated or malignant hypertension is present when funduscopy shows bilateral hemorrhages, which tend to be flame-shaped or linear, and diastolic blood pressure is >120 mmHg. In the days before effective drug treatment of hypertension, around 80% of patients with malignant hypertension died within a year. Blurred vision is a common presenting complaint; other symptoms include morning headaches which tend to be occipital, exertional dyspnea, and weight loss. Bleeding, such as epistaxis or hemospermia, may occur. Earlier and more effective treatment of hypertension has rendered encephalopathy with obtundation and seizures very rare, although the condition is still seen in children and in parts of Africa where malignant hypertension remains a major problem.

Papilledema results from a rise in intracranial pressure but, in itself, does not appear to identify patients with a prognosis that is significantly different from those who have retinal hemorrhages and 'cottonwool' spots. A diagnosis of malignant hypertension cannot be sustained if hemorrhages are unilateral because of the possibility of confusion with central or branch retinal vein occlusion. Magnetic resonance scanning of the brain often demonstrates deep white matter edema in the parieto-occipital region, so-called posterior leuko-encephalopathy.

Cottonwool spots, or soft exudates, are areas of infarction of the nerve fiber layer of the retina. In contrast, refractile 'hard exudates' are caused by the escape of plasma from permeable small vessels with deposition of lipid in the retina. Hard exudates tend to cluster at the macula and may give rise to an appearance described as a macular 'star', especially in the resolving phase of hypertensive retinopathy. Hemorrhages, cottonwool spots, and papilledema clear after only a few weeks of antihypertensive therapy, but hard exudates may persist for several months.

Hypertension causes narrowing of the retinal arterioles, which may show focal spasm in more severe cases. The normal ratio of artery : vein diameter is more than 3 : 4. Changes in the light reflex reflect hyalinization of the vessel wall or arteriosclerosis, and occur with hypertension and increasing age; grading is difficult in clinical practice. More severe grades of high blood pressure cause 'silver wiring' of the arterioles, accompanied by right-angled crossing of veins by arterioles and 'nipping' of the retinal veins.

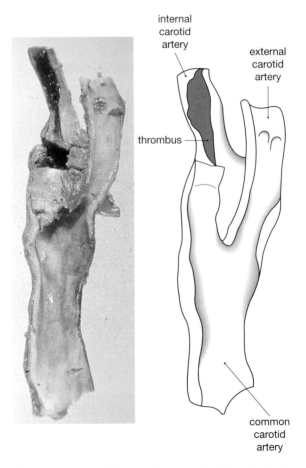

Figure 6 Postmortem section of the carotid artery at the bifurcation showing considerable atheroma in the internal carotid artery. The artery is occluded by thrombus

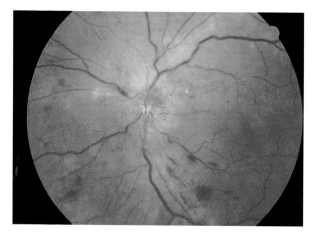

Figure 7 Funduscopy of a patient with malignant hypertension showing linear or flame-shaped retinal hemorrhages and papilledema. For a clinical diagnosis of malignant hypertension, such hemorrhages must be present in both eyes

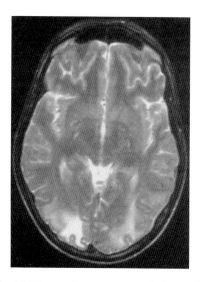

Figure 8 T2-weighted MRI scan showing posterior leukoencephalopathy or white matter edema in a man with malignant hypertension. The condition is reversible and has symptoms of headache, drowsiness, visual symptoms, and seizures

Heart

Left ventricular hypertrophy

An increase in peripheral vascular resistance is characteristic of the established phase of hypertension. Left ventricular work is increased as a consequence and results in concentric hypertrophy. Although changes in cardiac geometry tend to normalize wall stresses during systole, they reduce compliance, causing diastolic dysfunction, and increased myocardial oxygen demand.

A hypertrophic ventricle initially functions well but, in the later stages, there is progressive dilatation associated with a steep decline in performance. Subendocardial myocardial ischemia may be caused by the combined effects of poor perfusion due to diastolic dysfunction and increased demand for oxygen from hypertrophied myocytes. There is usually an accompanying reduction in capillary density or rarefaction and an increase in the diffusion distance for oxygen. Coronary flow reserve, which is the difference between normal flow rate and flow rate

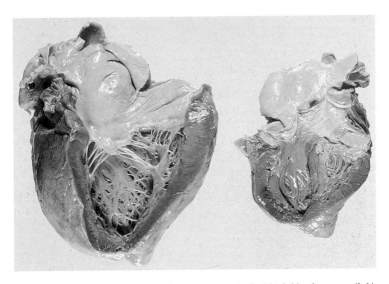

Figure 9 Coronal section of a heart from a patient who had high blood pressure (left) compared with a normal heart (right). Note the increase in the overall size of the hypertensive heart and in the thickness of the left ventricular wall

at maximum dilatation, is reduced in the hypertrophied ventricle. Patients with severe left ventricular hypertrophy are vulnerable to diastolic heart failure in the presence of cardiac arrhythmias and/or increased peripheral vascular resistance.

Part of the reduction in compliance of the left ventricle in hypertension is caused by deposition of increased collagen which may not be reversed by antihypertensive treatment. The hypertrophied left ventricle becomes stiff and may not be adequately filled during diastole. Thus, a serious decline in cardiac output may ensue if atrial fibrillation removes the active phase of ventricular filling. Echocardiography is considerably more sensitive than electrocardiography in detecting ventricular hypertrophy in hypertension, but magnetic resonance imaging is even better.

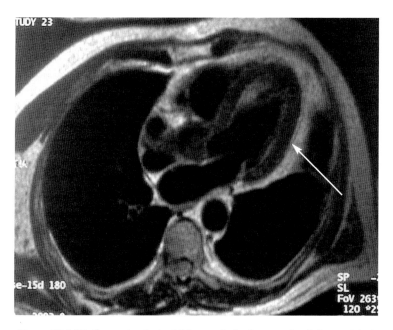

Figure 10 MRI (long-axis view) of left ventricular hypertrophy (left ventricle is arrowed) in a middle-aged patient with resistant hypertension. The hypertrophy is concentric and the leaflets of the mitral valve can be clearly seen below and to the left. MRI is probably superior to echocardiography in quantifying ventricular hypertrophy

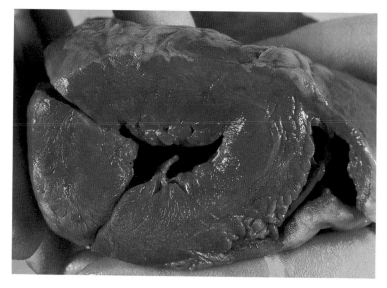

Figure 11 Transverse section of a heart in chronic severe hypertension shows marked left ventricular failure

Severe left ventricular hypertrophy predisposes to serious ventricular arrhythmias and sudden death. The Framingham Study has shown that left ventricular hypertrophy is an independent risk factor. During 12 years of follow-up, the mortality of patients with left ventricular hypertrophy, as determined by electrocardiographic criteria, was 16%, rising to 60% in the presence of a concurrent 'strain pattern'.

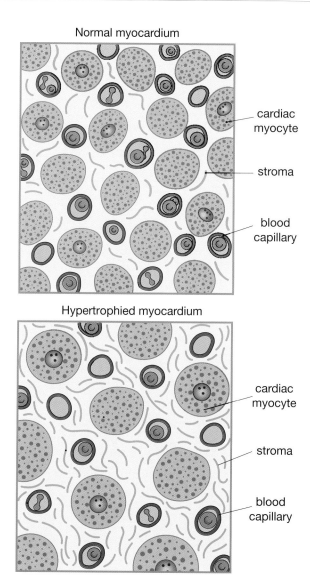

Figure 12 Schematic diagrams showing the typical appearances of normal (top) compared with hypertrophied (bottom) myocardium

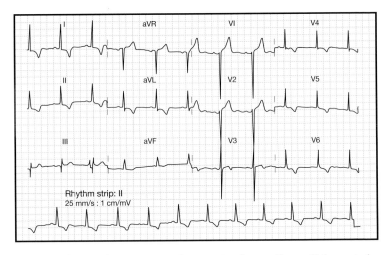

Figure 13 Electrocardiogram in severe hypertension shows evidence of left ventricular failure by limb- and chest-lead voltage criteria. There is ST-segment depression in the lateral leads, described as the 'strain' pattern. The usual chest-lead criterion for left ventricular failure is: S wave in V1 + R wave in V5 > 35mm. Criteria in limb-leads are: R wave in V1 + S wave in V3 > 25 mm or R wave in lead 1 > 12 mm

Coronary artery disease

In Europe and North America, high blood pressure is also a major factor for coronary artery disease and sudden cardiac death. As with stroke, the relationship between blood pressure and coronary events is probably continuous across the whole blood pressure distribution. Thus, those in the highest quintile of the distribution have an incidence about five times greater than those in the lowest quintile. The event rate in the lowest part of the distribution is generally rather low and variable between studies. The earlier proposal that low diastolic blood pressure in treated hypertension precipitates coronary events is not supported by the results of the Hypertension Optimal Treatment (HOT) Study.

High blood pressure accelerates the development of atherosclerosis, which is also highly dependent on blood levels of cholesterol, LDL cholesterol, and other lipoproteins, such as lipoprotein(a), as well as cigarette smoking, obesity and diabetes mellitus. In Japan and China, where populations have low cholesterol levels, the incidence of coronary artery disease is relatively low, although the stroke mortality rate in China is currently around twice that in the United Kingdom.

Few individual trials of drug treatment of hypertension have shown significant reductions in myocardial infarction or coronary events, but meta-analysis does show a significant overall benefit. Drug treatments appear to reduce slightly the incidence of congestive heart failure, probably as a reflection of the prevention or reversal of left ventricular hypertrophy. There is preliminary evidence that the decline in cognitive function may be prevented by antihypertensive therapy in patients who have had strokes, and a little evidence that treatment of elderly patients with hypertension may reduce the incidence of dementia.

Various explanations for the failure to completely reverse the risk of coronary events have been proposed. For example, it is possible that the time course of the effects of lowering blood pressure on atherosclerosis is different from the time course of small-vessel disease. Indeed, most treatment trials have been of relatively short duration (3–5 years) and have terminated at the point where a significant reduction in stroke is attained. Meta-analysis of the results of all the major trials of treatment in mild-to-moderate hypertension suggests a significant reduction in coronary event rate of about 14%. One major randomized controlled trial, ALLHAT, has compared the incidence of fatal coronary disease and non-fatal myocardial infarction in over 33 000 patients with hypertension and a high risk of coronary disease. There were no significant differences between treatment with a thiazide diuretic, dihydropyridine calcium antagonist and angiotensin-converting enzyme inhibitor.

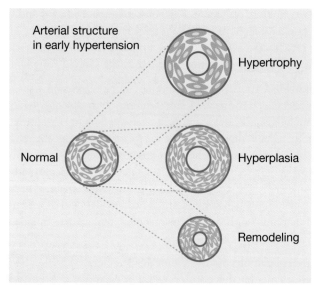

Figure 14 Schematic diagram showing three types of thickening of the media in resistance arterioles caused by hypertension. Such thickening results in an increase in wall : lumen ratio

Aorta and arteries

In hypertension, the small arteries develop medial thickening and arteriosclerosis is accelerated. The change in small-vessel geometry results in an increase in wall-to-wall lumen ratio (Figure 14) and enhances the pressor response to vasoconstrictor substances. This is often described as the 'vascular amplifier' and may have a role in aggravating hypertension. The possible causes of a change in wall-to-lumen ratio are smooth muscle hypertrophy, hyperplasia or rearrangement of the same cells around a reduced lumen, described as remodeling. In hypertension in humans, remodeling may predominate, but the relative importance of the three factors remains the subject of debate.

Circulating or local vasoactive agents such as angiotensin II also have growth-promoting effects on smooth muscle and, conversely, growth factors such as platelet-derived growth factor (PDGF) may be potent

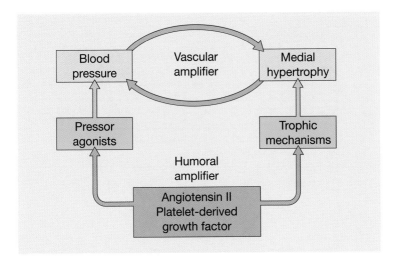

Figure 15 Schematic diagram of the humoral amplifier showing the pathways by which local and circulating vasoconstrictors may also promote medical hypertrophy

vasoconstrictors. This so-called humoral amplifier (Figure 15) may act in concert with the vascular amplifier to promote structural change. In contrast, vasodilators such as nitric oxide usually inhibit cell growth, and may reduce pressure by both direct and indirect mechanisms. Arterial structure is affected by local and circulating factors, and it has become increasingly evident that the vascular endothelium responds to hemodynamic stimuli by producing vasoactive substances, some of which also modulate smooth muscle cell growth.

Medial hypertrophy evolves towards arteriosclerosis, including so-called 'hyaline' sclerosis of arterioles as well as sclerosis of larger arteries. Age-related changes resemble those seen in long-standing hypertension. Hyalin is restricted to arterioles and the smallest arteries, and is concentrated in vessels of the kidney, brain, retina, spleen and gut with relative sparing of heart, skeletal muscle and skin.

In the brain, heart and kidneys, blood flow remains constant despite wide variations in arterial pressure, a phenomenon known as autoregulation (Figure 16). In hypertension, loss of arterial compliance due to

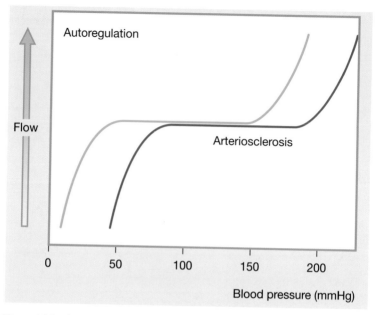

Figure 16 In the cerebral and renal circulations, auto-regulation maintains constant blood flow over a range of pressures. Arteriosclerosis due to hypertension or aging causes a shift of the autoregulatory curve to the right. As a consequence, the risk of cerebral and renal underperfusion during hypotension is increased, although susceptibility to malignant-phase hypertension is reduced

arteriosclerosis causes the autoregulation curve to be shifted to the right so that vasodilatation and 'flow reserve' are compromised.

In the aorta and other large elastic arteries, hypertension and aging cause dilatation, lengthening and loss of compliance. Unfolding of the ascending aorta is often seen on plain chest radiography and severe dilatation of the aortic root sometimes causes aortic regurgitation. Loss of elasticity accounts for the relatively greater increase of systolic blood pressure rather than diastolic blood pressure with age, and causes pulse-wave velocity to increase. The effect of this increased velocity is that the reflected wave from the periphery reaches the heart in systole rather than in diastole, thereby increasing cardiac workload and

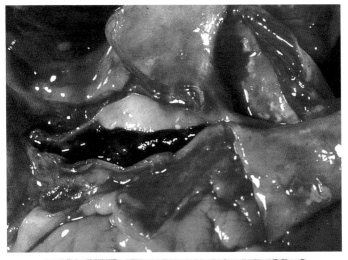

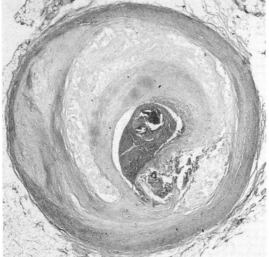

Figure 17 Recent thrombus can be seen at the origin of the right coronary artery close to the aorta (upper). Histology of a severely atheromatous coronary artery (lower) shows residual media (deep pink-staining). The artery is narrowed by atheromatous plaque comprising a mixture of pale fibrous tissue and clear lipid material. The plaque cap has ruptured, causing hemorrhage into the plaque and thrombosis of the lumen (H & E)

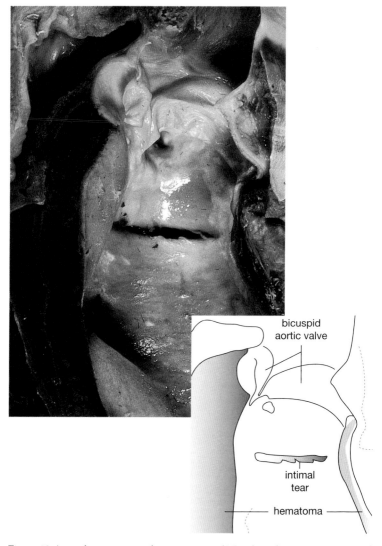

Figure 18 Aorta showing a typical transverse tear (2.5 cm) on the inner aspect around 3 cm above the aortic valve, the site of initiation of around 60 % of cases of aortic dissection. Hematoma can be seen on the inner surface of the vessel. Hypertension is the most common factor predisposing to aortic dissection

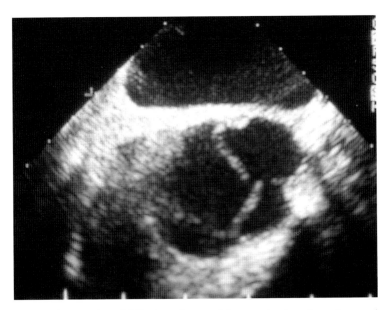

Figure 19 Transesophageal 2-D echocardiogram of the aorta showing a flap and tear, and a false lumen which probably contains thrombus. Color Doppler imaging (CDI) showed lower flow velocities in the false, compared with the true, lumen.

promoting ventricular hypertrophy. It is now clear that isolated systolic hypertension in the elderly benefits from treatment with antihypertensive drugs, especially diuretic-based regimens, but also with beta-blockers. Severe hypertension also causes an increase in glycosaminoglycan in the aortic media and predisposes to the relatively rare complication of aortic dissection (Figure 18).

Kidneys

Renal failure often develops in patients with malignant hypertension, but is relatively rare in non-malignant hypertension, perhaps because of more effective treatment. In the era before antihypertensive drugs, death from renal failure in malignant hypertension was commonplace. African–Americans have a high prevalence of renal impairment caused by hypertension, compared with Caucasians.

Malignant hypertension causes fibrinoid necrosis of the small arteries and arterioles in the kidney, especially in the afferent glomerular arterioles, but also affecting small radial arteries. Fibrin in the vessel wall is the result of plasmatic vasculosis, a process which allows plasma proteins, including fibrinogen, to gain access to the media (Figure 20). This is accompanied by necrosis of smooth muscle cells and thrombosis of the lumen, leading to obliteration of the glomeruli, and the presence of red cells and red casts in the urine. Intimal proliferation, which is most prominent in the radial arteries, leads to the characteristic 'onion-skin' appearance, which may represent a healing response to endothelial cell injury. The glomeruli undergo focal necrosis, and glomerular capillaries may rupture into Bowman's space and the renal tubules, to cause a 'flea-bitten' appearance to the surface of the kidney (Figure 21). Fibrin deposition in blood vessels occasionally causes fragmentation of circulating red blood cells, resulting in so-called microangiopathic hemolytic anemia with thrombocytopenia.

Lowering arterial pressure usually stabilizes renal function if renal impairment is due to hypertensive nephrosclerosis, and also reduces the rate of functional deterioration in many chronic renal conditions. The cause of progressive renal failure in kidney disease is still not well understood, although overperfusion of the reduced number of residual nephrons has been proposed as a pathogenetic mechanism.

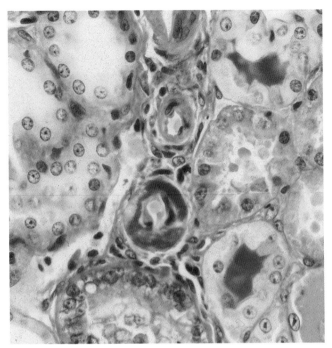

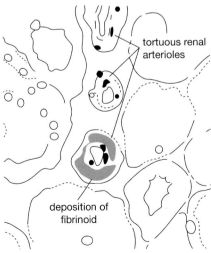

tortuous renal arterioles

deposition of fibrinoid

Figure 20 Histology of a kidney in severe hypertension showing red-staining 'fibrinoid' deposition in the media of an arteriole, a result of insudation of plasma proteins such as fibrinogen and fibrin. Proteins gain entry because vascular permeability is increased in response to damage caused by high intraluminal pressures (Martius scarlet-blue)

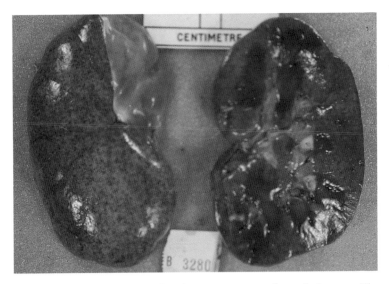

Figure 21 Kidneys in malignant-phase hypertension are swollen and edematous. The renal capsule has been removed to show the tiny punctate hemorrhages on the surface characteristic of the so-called 'flea-bitten' kidney

Diabetes mellitus

Diabetic nephropathy is a major cause of end-stage renal disease in the developed countries, with an average survival after the onset of persistent proteinuria of only 5–10 years. Treatment of hypertension slows the rate of loss of renal function and ACE inhibitors and angiotensin receptor antagonists appear to be more effective in this context than beta-blockers or the dihydropyridine calcium antagonists, perhaps because of specific effects on glomerular hemodynamics. In type I (insulin-dependent) diabetes, hypertension tends to develop in parallel with nephropathy and then promotes proteinuria and accelerates deterioration of renal function. Treatment with ACE inhibitors and angiotensin-1 receptor blockers clearly reduces proteinuria. Non-dihydropyridine calcium antagonists, such as verapamil, may have similar effects, but the evidence is less compelling. Optimal treatment of hypertension in diabetes is achieved at arterial pressures lower than in non-diabetics, so that target pressures should be set at < 140/80 mmHg, rather than at < 140/85 mmHg as non-diabetics.

Other aspects of treatment, such as more intensive control of blood sugar, also reduce the risk of developing micro- or macroalbuminuria. This was best demonstrated in the Diabetes Control and Complication Trial. In a few patients with more advance renal impairment due to diabetic nephropathy, there is an increased risk of renovascular disease so that ACE inhibitors have the potential to impair function.

In type II (non-insulin-dependent) diabetes, the relationship with hypertension may be somewhat different. It is clear from many epidemiological surveys that there is an association between hypertension, obesity, insulin resistance, and type II diabetes that is independent of nephropathy. Up to 25% of patients with type II diabetes develop microalbuminuria. Hypertension worsens proteinuria and accelerates renal impairment. As in type I diabetes, microalbuminuria as well as arterial pressures may be an indication for treatment. The presence of diabetes is a factor in the choice of antihypertensive drug. There is evidence that, in patients with left ventricular hypertrophy, ACE inhibitors and angiotensin-1 receptor blockers are more effective than beta-blockers and may be usefully combined with low-dose thiazide diuretics.

Measurement of blood pressure

For routine clinical purposes, the mercury sphygmomanometer (Figure 22) remains a robust, reliable and accurate instrument for measurement of arterial pressure. Aneroid devices tend to be less reliable and should be checked at least once a year against a mercury instrument. Such a check is conveniently made using a 'Y' connection between the tubing of the two instruments. There is now a wide variety of electronic machines available for home blood pressure monitoring, although the standards of accuracy vary considerably. Equipment validated by robust protocols, such as outlined by the British Hypertension Society, is preferred.

Accuracy

There are important points to observe if accurate measurements are to be obtained by indirect methods. The first is the vexed question of cuff size, which has exercised minds since Riva Rocci described the first instrument in 1896. Cuffs that are too small overestimate pressure and the converse is also true. There is general agreement that the bladder should almost encircle the arm and have a width that is 40% of the circumference of the arm. Current recommendations in the UK are to use a 22 x 12.5 cm cuff for adults with 35–42 cm arm circumferences. With arm circumferences < 35 cm, a smaller bladder (18 x 18 cm) should be used and for arms > 47 cm in circumference, a longer 12 x 40 cm or longer and wider 16 x 40 cm cuff should be chosen.

It has become apparent that training in the correct use of the mercury sphygmomanometer is essential to reduce error. In previous years, instruction was often minimal. Methods of reducing observer error include formal instruction combined with the use of videos, films or audiocassette tapes.

Mercury sphygmomanometers should be checked every 6 months in hospital use and every year otherwise. Problems are relatively

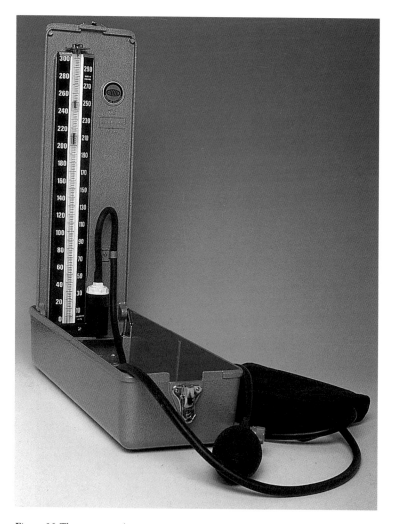

Figure 22 The mercury sphygmomanometer remains the standard instrument for measurement of blood pressure. Common remedial causes of inaccuracy are: the mercury meniscus does not start at zero; the inside of the glass tube is black; and the valve is not functioning properly. It should be possible to adjust the rate of descent of the mercury meniscus to 2 mm/s or less

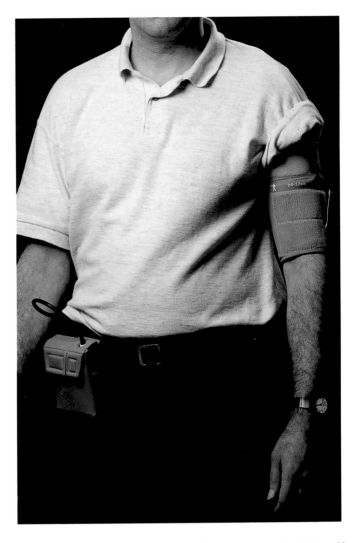

Figure 23 Contemporary equipment for the indirect measurement of ambulatory blood pressures

infrequent, but include loss of mercury so that the meniscus is not at zero when the cuff is deflated, and black deposits of oxidized mercury on the inner surface of the glass that obscure the meniscus. Occasionally, there is a leak in the system so that the rate of descent of the column of mercury is > 2 mm/s. It should always be possible to inflate the bladder to a pressure > 200 mmHg in less than 5 seconds. The Velcro on a cuff may wear out so that there is poor apposition of bladder to arm.

Measurements of pressure should be made with the arm supported at heart level. At the initial clinical assessment of a patient, blood pressures should be measured in both arms sequentially. If the difference between the arms is > 20/10 mmHg, then simultaneous measurements of both arms using two instruments should be taken and the arm that gives the higher values should be used for subsequent monitoring. In patients in the last trimester of pregnancy, in the recumbent position, there is an increase in pulse rate and narrowing of the pulse pressure due to sympathetic activation caused by reduced venous return. Placing the patient in the lateral position minimizes the reflex activation.

Blood pressures are normally recorded to the nearest 2 mmHg. In most circumstances, the diastolic blood pressure is measured at Korotkoff phase V, the point at which sounds disappear. In cases where there is a wide pulse pressure due to aortic regurgitation or rapid run-off into the peripheral circulation, phase V may continue to 0 mmHg. In such an event, the diastolic blood pressure should be recorded at phase IV, where there is muffling of the heart sounds reported.

Ambulatory monitoring

Non-invasive ambulatory monitoring of blood pressure is available for diagnosis and assessment of the adequacy of control of hypertension and antihypertensive treatment (Figure 23). The technique provides a profile of blood pressures over 24 or 48 hours, with information on diurnal patterns and nocturnal levels of blood pressure. There is not yet sufficient epidemiological data to relate levels to morbidity and mortality. At present, normal values tend to be defined on the basis of cross-sectional studies and meta-analyses. It has been proposed that normal daytime values may be as low as 126/88 or as high as 150/95 mmHg.

The technique has value in detecting 'white coat' hypertension and identifying those who do not show a nocturnal dip in pressure. The white coat effect may be a factor in 20% or more of patients with hypertension diagnosed by office or clinic blood pressure recording. It has further been proposed that the term 'white coat' hypertension should be reserved for patients who have persistently high clinic blood pressure readings, but normal ambulatory values, whereas the term 'white coat phenomenon' can be reserved for those who have a tendency for higher values during the first 1–2 hours of ambulatory recording (Figure 24). It has also not yet been ascertained that white coat hypertension has an entirely benign prognosis. What is well established is that the correlation between ambulatory blood pressure and left ventricular hypertrophy is closer with ambulatory than with office recordings and, thus, the technique is useful in patients who have borderline hypertension (Figure 25).

On occasions, ambulatory monitoring has been useful in detecting fluctuating hypertension in pheochromocytoma, and a lack of diurnal variation sometimes points to a secondary cause. In patients with high clinic recordings despite treatment, ambulatory recordings may demonstrate whether blood pressure control is truly poor. Blood pressure profile changes over 24 hours also provide insights into antihypertensive drug effects and facilitate calculation of trough-to-peak ratios for individual agents.

The issue of accuracy is pertinent and, thus, it is essential that the instruments available on the market should meet validation criteria such as the British Hypertension Society protocol. General experience suggests that accuracy is not maintained at high levels of blood pressure, although the practical significance of this type of error is likely to be minimal. At present, the ambulatory systems make only intermittent measurements of pressure. Although more detailed and accurate profiles can be obtained by intra-arterial methods, their invasive nature excludes them from routine practice. It is already clear that ambulatory measurements are superior to clinic values in terms of prognosis.

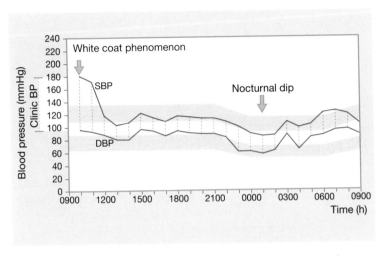

Figure 24 Pattern of 24-h ambulatory blood pressures in a patient with white-coat hypertension. Clinic blood pressure was 182/96 mmHg, but the mean 24-h pressure was only 109/81 mmHg

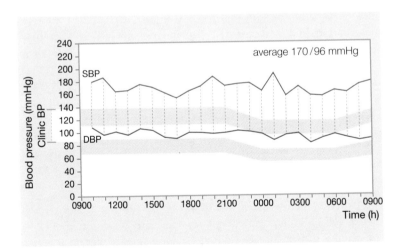

Figure 25 These 24-h ambulatory blood pressures are higher than the clinic pressure, which was 148/86 mmHg. There is no nocturnal dip. Ambulatory pressures are better predictors of left ventricular hypertrophy than are clinic measurements

Investigation of secondary hypertension

Renovascular disease

Renovascular disease is generally uncommon if sought in asymptomatic patients with mild to moderate hypertension. The prevalence in cross-sectional surveys in developed countries is usually around 3% or less. Certain groups are at high risk of atheromatous renal artery stenosis, notably patients with peripheral vascular disease, wherein approximately 30% of patients have unilateral, and around 10% have bilateral, renal artery stenosis. Bilateral disease may comprise stenosis on one side and an occlusion contralaterally. With stenosis of more than 75% of the luminal diameter, there is a risk of arterial occlusion, ranging from 8% to 16% over 2–3 years.

Deterioration of renal function after treatment with ACE inhibitors or angiotensin receptor antagonists is now a relatively common cause of presentation and non-steroidal anti-inflammatory drugs can have similar effects. Renovascular disease may also be suspected where there is an unexplained deterioration in control of blood pressure with drug treatment, especially if such treatment does not include an ACE inhibitor or angiotensin receptor antagonist. If there is peripheral vascular disease or abdominal aortic aneurysm, there is quite often concurrent significant renal artery stenosis. Although not often encountered nowadays, patients with malignant or accelerated hypertension are also more likely to have renovascular disease, especially if the condition develops in a patient > 50 years old.

For patients < 40 years of age, renovascular disease is uncommon except with fibromuscular dysplasia. This rare condition should be suspected if a woman, especially a cigarette-smoker, develops severe hypertension with no family history of high blood pressure or stroke. Plasma renin activity is usually high in the untreated state and normalization of blood pressure after treatment with an ACE inhibitor

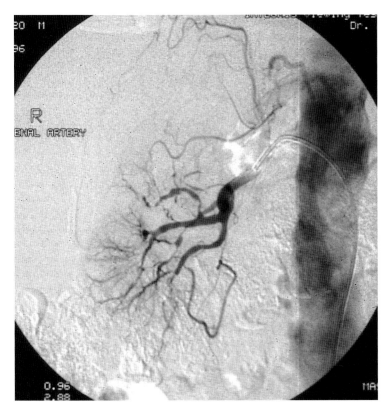

Figure 26 Digital subtraction arteriogram of a kidney from a patient with renal impairment caused by longstanding hypertension. The architecture of the intrarenal arteries is highly abnormal, and there is rarefaction, pruning and variation in arterial caliber

or angiotensin receptor antagonist is characteristic. The typical appearances are relatively easy to identify on angiography, and there may be a 'beaded' segment of artery where areas of arterial narrowing are interspersed with areas of dilatation. Other arteries of similar caliber, such as the carotid or mesenteric artery, may be affected. The condition predisposes to arterial dissection which, in the case of the renal artery, may present with flank pain and hematuria.

Fibromuscular disease responds particularly well to revascularization by angioplasty or surgery, providing that technical success has been achieved. Blood pressures are normalized in more than 50% of cases. This contrasts with the response rate in atheromatous renal artery disease where cure occurs in less than 20% of patients treated. As with most forms of hypertension, the factors which tend to predict a poor blood pressure response to revascularization include overall impairment of renal function, reduced kidney size and long-term hypertension.

The low prevalence of renovascular disease in the general hypertensive population at around 3% indicates that screening tests must have a high degree of both sensitivity and specificity. The best functional tests available miss around 30% of cases and give positive yield on arteriography of approximately one in five cases. Of the functional tests available, rapid-sequence intravenous urography is now obsolete. Measurement of plasma renin activity 1 hour after administration of captopril has a sensitivity of 84% and a specificity of 93%, but is often compromised by prior antihypertensive drug treatment.

Magnetic resonance angiography and spiral computed tomography (CT) are the imaging modalities of choice. Renal scintigraphy after captopril was once the best non-invasive screening method, but diethylene-triamine pentaacetic acid (DTPA) scintigraphy has a sensitivity of only 70–80% with a 90% specificity, and the widely used mercaptoacetyl triglycine (MAG-3) technique is probably less sensitive. Doppler ultrasonography of the main renal arteries with contrast is sometimes useful, but is highly operator-dependent. Around 8% of arteries may not be visualized and approximately 20% of kidneys are supplied by more than one artery. Pulsatility of an interlobar artery distal to stenosis, measured by Doppler technology, is inadequate for screening, although it may be useful in detecting restenosis after angioplasty.

Some centers, including that of the author, only screen those patients in whom there is a high index of clinical suspicion. Intra-arterial digital subtraction angiography, using a 4-F catheter and an aortic flush injection of contrast, is the best means of visualizing a renal artery

Right renal artery stenosis   Left renal artery stenosis

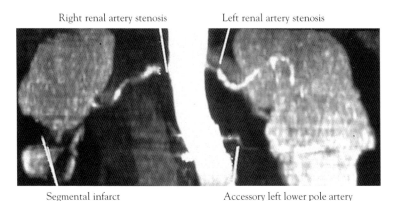

Segmental infarct   Accessory left lower pole artery

Figure 27 Maximum-intensity projection of a spiral CT angiogram showing bilateral renal artery stenosis and infarction of the lower pole of the right kidney

stenosis and is usually performed at the time of revascularization. Intravenous injection methods require larger doses of contrast and adequate definition of the renal arteries may not be attained, especially in cases where there is poor left ventricular function. Renal vein renin sampling after captopril stimulation is occasionally useful in diagnosis.

Surgery for renal artery stenosis has been largely superseded by percutaneous balloon angioplasty. Endovascular stents allow treatment of ostial lesions and cases where elastic recoil is a problem. However, a randomized trial from The Netherlands of balloon angioplasty in 106 patients with hypertension and atherosclerotic renal artery stenosis showed no benefit, compared with medical treatment, in terms of arterial pressures or renal function. The restenosis rate at 1 year was almost 50%. Few patients in this trial were treated with placement of a stent and at least one further trial is underway (ASTRAL). There have also been occasional case reports of beneficial effects of treating renal artery stenosis in patients with heart failure.

The complication rate of angioplasty and stent placement in experienced hands is low, although 5–10% of cases may develop groin hematoma. Arteriography or angioplasty in patients with severe

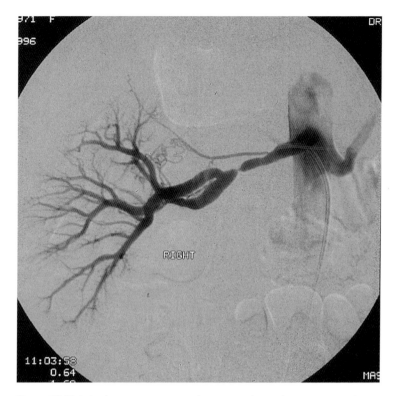

Figure 28 Digital subtraction angiogram showing a tight renal artery stenosis due to localized fibromuscular dysplasia in a 27-year-old nurse who had hypertension. Longer stenotic segments often present with a 'string-of-beads' appearance

atherosclerosis may precipitate cholesterol embolism which can result in deterioration in renal function, abdominal pain, livedo reticularis or ischemic lesions of the toes.

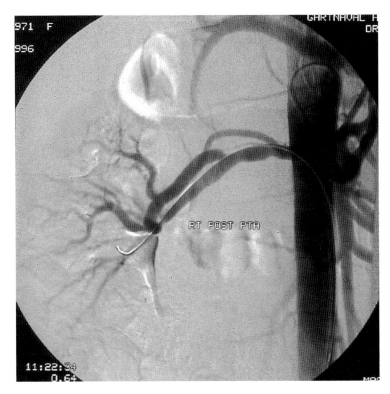

Figure 29 Digital subtraction angiogram of the same artery as in Figure 28 shown after successful percutaneous balloon angioplasty

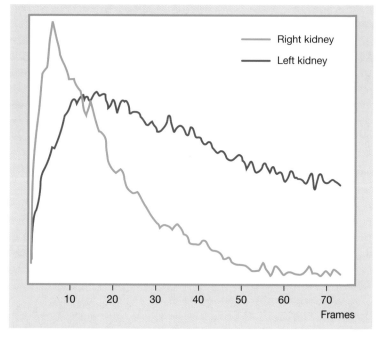

Figure 30 Graph showing typical curves derived by captopril renography of a patient with left renal artery stenosis. The $t_{1/2}$ and t_{max} are characteristically prolonged. The method is useful for detecting unilateral functional renal artery stenosis

Renal hypertension

Most renal diseases that impair kidney function cause high blood pressure. Patients with hypertension while undergoing renal replacement treatment often have left ventricular hypertrophy.

The type of glomerulonephritis that is most often encountered in blood pressure clinics is IgA nephropathy or Berger's disease. The condition is so-called because immunocytochemistry of renal tissue shows that mesangial deposition of IgA is a prominent feature. The disease appears to be ubiquitous, but is perhaps less common in Northern Europe and the USA than in Southern Europe and Asia. Children present with frank hematuria in association with respiratory failure, but hypertension associated with persistent microscopic hematuria and mild proteinuria may bring the condition to the attention of physicians treating hypertension. The condition tends to affect men and progression to end-stage renal failure may be relatively slow.

Most patients with chronic renal failure have high blood pressure caused largely by a combination of volume expansion due to retention of sodium and water, and activation of the renin–angiotensin system. Control of blood pressure often necessitates multiple-drug regimens, including loop diuretics such as frusemide, which may need to be given in large doses. Restriction of dietary sodium intake to around 50 mmol/day or less may be a helpful measure.

In patients undergoing dialysis treatment, blood pressure control is more readily achieved with the continuous ambulatory peritoneal technique than with intermittent peritoneal dialysis or hemodialysis. Erythropoietin treatment of anemia tends to increase arterial pressure in parallel with the rise in hematocrit and blood viscosity.

Chronic renal disease is the most common cause of high blood pressure in children and young adults. Reflux nephropathy is a particularly important cause of high blood pressure in women of this age group and may present as severe or malignant hypertension. Disease is often bilateral, but unilateral reflux with renal scarring is sometimes seen. Hypertension may be cured or greatly improved by nephrectomy, provided that there is adequate function in the remaining kidney. High arterial pressures seem to be found quite early in patients with autosomal dominant polycystic kidney disease. Mild high blood pressure in children or young adults may be due to primary hypertension, but investigation to exclude renal disease is often appropriate in this age group. The rate of rise in blood pressure in adolescents is particularly marked in the overweight.

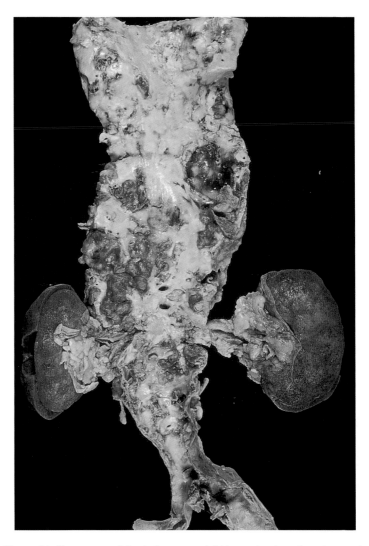

Figure 31 Postmortem abdominal aorta and kidneys showing ulcerating aortic atheroma, which may cause cholesterol embolism in life. Clinical manifestations of cholesterol embolism include renal impairment, livido reticularis and ischemic areas in the toes

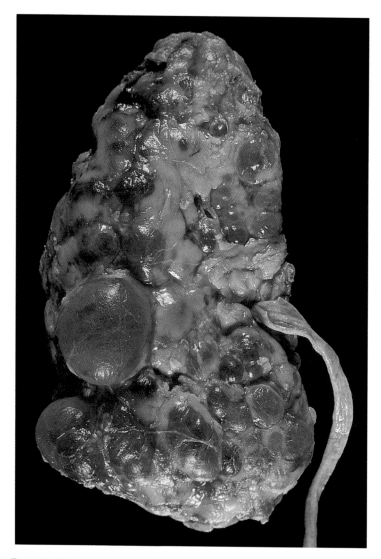

Figure 32 Kidney in autosomal dominant (adult) polycystic kidney disease showing large cysts which have replaced normal kidney tissue

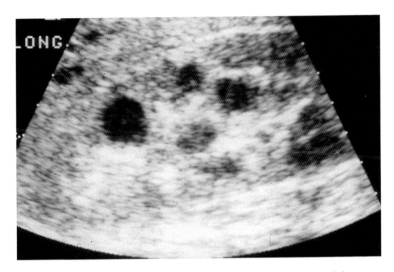

Figure 33 Ultrasonogram (longitudinal view) of a kidney with autosomal dominant polycystic kidney disease shows an enlarged and cystic right kidney. There is little likelihood of the condition if an ultrasound study in early adulthood is negative. The genetic abnormality associated with the most common form of the disease, designated PKDI, has been localized to the short arm of chromosome 16

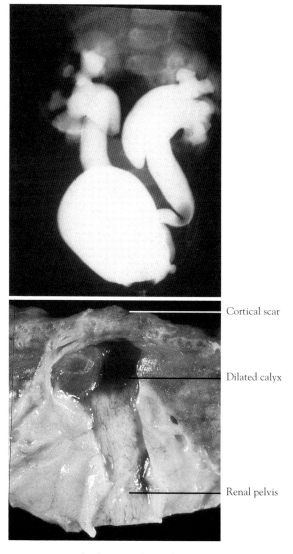

Cortical scar

Dilated calyx

Renal pelvis

Figure 34 Micturating cystogram (top) in an infant with severe vesicoureteric reflux shows intrarenal reflux in the upper poles of the kidneys. In the postmortem specimen (bottom), one of the dilated calyces shows loss of the overlying parenchyma

Mineralocorticoid hypertension

Primary aldosteronism

Primary aldosteronism or Conn's syndrome is a much less common cause of high blood pressure than is renovascular hypertension. It most often affects women, and may present with symptoms of weakness and polyuria. The condition is usually first suspected after routine measurement of plasma electrolytes reveals concentrations indicative of hypokalemia, accompanied by a slight increase in the serum concentration of sodium. As hypokalemia may be intermittent, measurement of serum concentrations of potassium is not a good screening test, and serum potassium concentrations may be normal if dietary sodium intake is low.

Paralysis of skeletal muscle caused by severe hypokalemia is rare, but has been seen in patients who have primary aldosteronism after treatment with a thiazide or loop diuretic, and in subjects habituated to licorice.

In primary aldosteronism, there is a marked suppression of plasma renin activity or concentration except in patients treated with a diuretic or following a low sodium diet. As a screening test, renin levels tend to be non-specific because nearly 30% of white hypertensives and a higher proportion of blacks have somewhat low renin values. The confounding effect of a low sodium diet on aldosteronism may be excluded through measurement of urinary sodium excretion over 24 hours and relating this value to the concurrent activity of renin. Plasma renin activity remains suppressed after ACE inhibitor treatment, in contrast to primary hypertension.

A diagnosis of primary aldosteronism is confirmed by high plasma concentrations of aldosterone in samples taken in the morning or increased urinary aldosterone excretion with marked suppression of plasma renin activity and concentration. Some centers still use suppression tests with aldosterone measurement after sodium loading. An anomalous postural fall in plasma levels of aldosterone is sometimes present. In the presence of low levels of renin and angiotensin II, aldosterone secretion follows the diurnal rhythm of adrenocorticotropic hormone (ACTH) such that a component of the decrease

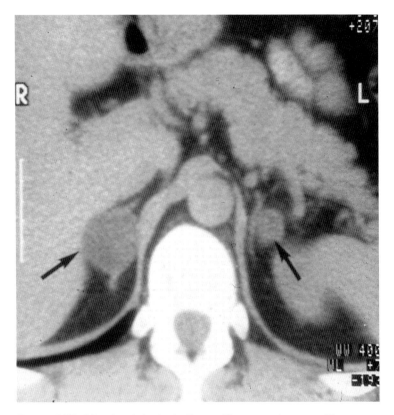

Figure 35 CT of the adrenal glands of a 40-year-old patient with primary aldosteronism showing bilateral tumors, a highly unusual finding as aldosteronomas are virtually always unilateral. In this case, aldosterone secretion was confined to the smaller lesion on the left, demonstrated by aldosterone levels in adrenal venous blood. The larger right-sided lesion had a slightly lower attenuation coefficient and was a non-functioning adenoma

observed after ambulation between 08.00 and 12.00 may be due to the diurnal variation in ACTH. Several centers now prefer to measure aldosterone/renin ratios as a screening test of primary aldosteronism, but the sensitivity and specificity of this approach are not completely defined. Prevalences of primary aldosteronism up to 10–15% are still claimed by some centers but the issue is debated. In cases of difficulty,

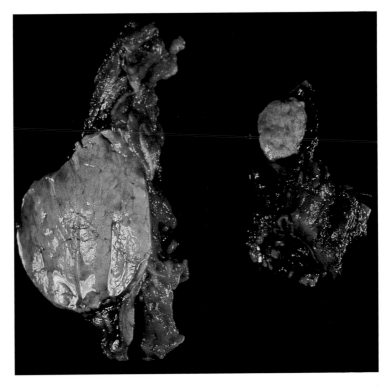

Figure 36 Resected adrenal tumors from the same patient as in Figure 35. Analysis of tumor steroid content demonstrated a high concentration of aldosterone only in the tumor on the left

measurement of the 10-hydroxycortisol steroids 18-hydroxycorticosterone and 18-hydroxycortisol may be helpful. Raised levels of 18-hydroxycortisol suggest autonomous secretion of aldosterone. Levels of the 18-hydroxylated steroids are less likely to be attenuated by hypokalemia compared with those of aldosterone.

Low plasma renin activity accompanied by low concentrations of aldosterone point to hypertension caused by another mineralocorticoid, either self-administered or endogenous. Some of the rare syndromes due to inherited deficiencies of the enzyme for corticosteroid biosynthesis cause mineralocorticoid hypertension with high levels of ACTH stimulating adrenal secretion of deoxycorticosterone.

Once a biochemical diagnosis of primary aldosteronism is established, localization of an adenoma is the next step. Tumors are often visualized on CT or MRI, but small adenomas < 1.5 cm in diameter may not be recognized. CT does not distinguish non-functioning adenomas from aldosteronomas. If a tumor > 3 cm in diameter is identified, then malignancy should be suspected. Malignant renal tumors seldom present with mineralocorticoid hypertension and rarely, if ever, synthesize aldosterone, but some secrete other mineralocorticoids, notably dexoycorticosterone.

If an adenoma is suspected, then adrenal vein catheterization with measurement of aldosterone in adrenal venous blood is the most accurate way of confirming or establishing the diagnosis before surgery. However, this may be difficult on the right side. A small proportion of patients (10–20%) have idiopathic aldosteronism without adenoma, although a tumor cannot be excluded unless adrenal venous sampling had been carried out. Differentiation of idiopathic aldosteronism from low renin primary hypertension can also be difficult.

The initial treatment of primary aldosteronism is with potassium-sparing diuretics. These include aldosterone antagonists such as spironolactone (doses of up to 300 mg/day) but amiloride (10–40 mg/day) may be used if there are drug side-effects such as gynecomastia. With spironolactone, there is a significant incidence of side-effects and there are concerns over the potential of long-term large doses to cause breast cancer. Epleronone is a recently introduced aldosterone antagonist which may have less estrogenic properties, but experience with this drug is currently limited. The response of blood pressure to drug treatment tends to predict the effect of surgery.

Plasma renin activity is a convenient index of extracellular fluid volume status during drug treatment and of the dose of amiloride or spironolactone. The dose that controls blood pressure to normal levels often reduces exchangeable sodium, measured by isotopic dilution, to below normal, which may reflect the relatively high prevalence of residual hypertension after surgery.

Blood pressure after surgery is normalized in only 50% of patients. If renal function is impaired, then a satisfactory blood pressure response to medical treatment or surgery is much less likely. Extracellular volume expansion due to mineralocorticoids normally causes an increase in glomerular filtration rate so that creatinine clearance tends to fall after medical or surgical treatment unless renal function is impaired.

Other forms of mineralocorticoid hypertension

Syndromes caused by deficiency of the enzymes involved in cortisol biosynthesis, such as 17α-hydroxylase and 11β-hydroxylase, cause mineralocorticoid hypertension. 17α-Hydroxylase deficiency is accompanied by failure of sexual development, as the enzyme is necessary for synthesis of sex steroids. 11β-Hydroxylase deficiency is accompanied by virilization in females or precocious puberty in males. In both syndromes, decreased cortisol secretion releases ACTH from feedback inhibition, resulting in excessive secretion of the mineralocorticoid deoxycorticosterone. A further rare enzyme deficiency is 11β-hydroxysteroid deficiency, wherein cortisol to cortisone metabolism within the kidney and other tissues is reduced, thereby exposing the mineralocorticoid receptor to cortisol in high concentrations. This 'shuttle' enzyme normally protects the mineralocorticoid receptor from circulating cortisol and is inhibited by licorice and the licorice derivative carbenoxolone sodium. Mineralocorticoid hypertension due to subunit mutation (beta or gamma) of the epithelial sodium channel downstream of the mineralocorticoid receptor causes Liddle's syndrome, when renin and aldosterone levels are suppressed and inheritance is autosomal dominant. A further autosomal dominant syndrome of hypertension caused by an abnormal mineralocorticoid receptor has recently been defined.

Cushing's syndrome

Hypertension also occurs frequently in Cushing's syndrome, although the mechanism is not as clearly defined as in primary aldosteronism. Hypertension appears to occur most often in ACTH-mediated disease. Several factors may be involved in the pathogenesis, including activation of type I (mineralocorticoid) and type II (glucocorticoid) receptors by cortisol, and production of other hypertensinogenic steroids from the adrenal cortex. Hypokalemia is more likely if ACTH levels are particularly high, as in the ectopic syndrome. Cushing's syndrome due to an adrenal adenoma or carcinoma is relatively uncommon and accounts for around 10% of cases.

Hypertension in pituitary-dependent Cushing's disease usually responds to transsphenoidal hypophysectomy. Otherwise, hypertensive inpatients with Cushing's syndrome should be treated with conventional antihypertensive drugs.

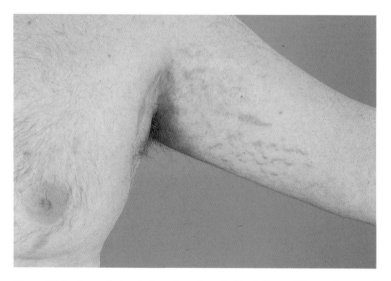

Figure 37 Axillary striae in pituitary-dependant Cushing's disease. The mechanism of the hypertension in Cushing's syndrome has not yet been completely ascertained. Hypokalemia is unusual except in cases with ectopic secretion of adrenocorticotropic hormone (ACTH), most usually from a carcinoid tumor

Pheochromocytoma

Pheochromocytoma is a rare cause of secondary hypertension which often causes problems in diagnosis. Routine screening in mild to moderate hypertension is not merited. Symptoms include paroxysmal headache, sweating and pallor. In some cases, hypertension may worsen with drug treatment especially if non-selective beta-blockers have been given.

Pheochromocytoma is often called the 'disease of 10%': around 10% are malignant, 10% are bilateral, and 10% are extra-adrenal. Bilateral disease is almost invariable in type IIA multiple endocrine neoplasia, a Mendelian-dominant condition caused by a mutation in the RET proto-oncogene and associated with medullary carcinoma of the thyroid. The less common variant is type IIB where there are associated mucosal neuromas and skeletal deformities. Genetic screening with DNA probes can now identify carriers with a high degree of confidence. The Mendelian-dominant von Hippel–Lindau disease also predisposes to pheochromocytoma and renal carcinoma.

Diagnosis is best made from measurements of plasma and urine concentrations of norepinephrine and epinephrine. Plasma levels of catecholamines are almost invariably raised if hypertension is present when samples are taken. Suppression tests with clonidine provide the most sensitive method of diagnosis and easily distinguish raised plasma levels of catecholamines due to sympathoadrenal activation from raised levels caused by autonomous tumor secretion. Plasma levels of chromogranin A or neuropeptide Y endothelin may be raised in pheochromocytoma, but have not found a role in routine diagnosis.

Tumors are usually located on MRI or CT; ultrasonography is not sensitive enough to detect small lesions. Catheterization and selective sampling from the inferior vena cava and left renal vein for catecholamines are seldom required. Approximately 80% of tumors take up radioiodine ^{131}I-labeled metaiodobenzylguanidine (MIBG), which may be helpful in scintigraphic localization of primary tumors and detection of metastatic deposits. Malignant tumors often metastasize to bone and isotope bone scans with an agent such as technetium 99m-labeled methylene diphosphonate should be routine before considering surgery. Some malignant tumors have been treated with

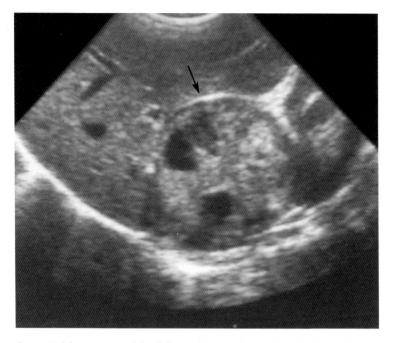

Figure 38 Ultrasonogram of the abdomen showing a large, right adrenal pheochromocytoma (arrowed) containing several fluid-filled areas

therapeutic doses of [^{131}I]MIBG and a few, less differentiated tumors have shown a useful response to cytotoxic drug treatment.

The long-acting non-competitive alpha-blocker phenoxybenzamine remains the drug of choice for controlling arterial pressure before surgery. Competitive blockers of the α_1 receptor have been somewhat disappointing in clinical practice. β_1-Adrenergic blockers may be used to control tachycardia. Most centers now use sodium nitroprusside for intraoperative control of blood pressure rather than the short-acting competitive blocker phentolamine, which has rather short-lived effects on blood pressure. Cardiac arrhythmias are generally prevented by adequate control of pressure, together with β-adrenoceptor antagonists.

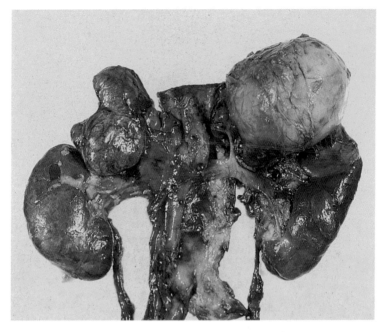

Figure 39 Bilateral adrenal pheochromocytomas due to multiple endocrine neoplasia type IIA, which has a Mendelian-dominant heritability and is caused by a mutation in the RET proto-oncogene. Gene carriers also develop medullary carcinoma of the thyroid

Hyperparathyroidism

There is an increased prevalence of hypertension in patients with primary hyperparathyroidism. Between 30% and 50% of affected patients have mild or moderately raised arterial pressure and some have left ventricular hypertrophy. The mechanism of the hypertension is not well understood, but may be related to the combined effects of extracellular hypercalcemia and excess parathyroid hormone.

The high blood pressure is not always corrected by parathyroid surgery, which may reflect an overlap with primary hypertension. In primary hypertension, a significant proportion of patients shows mild hypercalciuria and slightly raised levels of parathyroid hormone compared with controls that have normal blood pressure. This probably explains the increased incidence of renal calculus disease in patients with primary hypertension.

Acromegaly

Acromegaly is also associated with hypertension and there is some evidence that the hypertension is related to increased body sodium content. Hypertrophic changes in cardiac vascular muscle may also contribute to the raised blood pressures, which do not always respond to normalization of plasma levels of growth hormone.

Thyroid dysfunction

Hypothyroidism seems to cause a mild elevation of systolic and diastolic pressures by an undetermined mechanism.

Gestational hypertension

High blood pressure during pregnancy presents different problems. In normal pregnancy, blood pressure falls during the first trimester. Pre-eclamptic toxemia syndrome is diagnosed when hypertension with edema and proteinuria develops in late pregnancy associated with retardation of fetal growth. Thrombocytopenia and raised plasma concentrations of urate are characteristic, and intravascular volume is often reduced. In pre-eclampsia, blood pressures return to normal levels after delivery, but may occasionally persist a little longer.

In pregnancy-associated primary hypertension, high blood pressures are seen much earlier and pharmacological treatments seem to halve the risk of severe hypertension, although there is little evidence that pre-eclampsia is prevented. The evidence that one drug is better than others is poor and methyldopa and labetalol continue to be used.

Estrogens, oral contraceptives and hormone replacement therapy

The commonly used estrogen-containing oral contraceptives (which contain < 20 μg of estrogen) have mild pressor effects in many women. Therefore, monitoring of blood pressure before and after prescription is routine. A few subjects show a marked pressor response and are

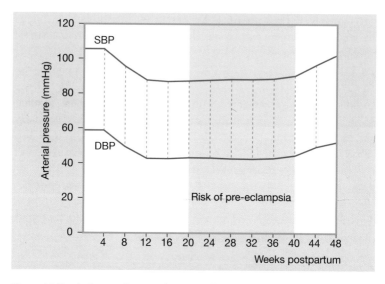

Figure 40 Graph showing the normal pattern of blood pressure in pregnancy. In the last trimester, lower values are obtained in the left lateral position. In the supine position, pressure from the gravid uterus on the inferior vena cava causes narrowing of the pulse pressure due to reflex activation of the sympathetic nervous system. Pre-eclampsia may develop at any time after week 20 of gestation. Early signs of the condition are hypertension and hyperuricemia followed by proteinuria, thrombocytopenia, hepatic dysfunction and placental impairment

probably patients who eventually go on to develop raised blood pressure in later life. The obsolete 50-μg preparations produced pressor effects that were more marked. Progestogen-only pills do not appear to raise blood pressure and may be prescribed in women with hypertension. Low-dose estrogen treatment given to women after the decline of ovarian estrogen secretion in menopause does not seem to raise blood pressure but use of estrogen and medroxyprogesterone in the Woman's Health Initiative randomized, controlled trial seemed to have a small adverse effect on development of breast cancer, stroke and cardiovascular events, with about 19 adverse events per 10 000 person-years exposure.

Coarctation of the aorta

Coarctation accounts for around 5–10% of all congenital cardiovascular anomalies and is a rare cause of hypertension. Aortic dissection, cerebral hemorrhage and heart failure are its associated complications.

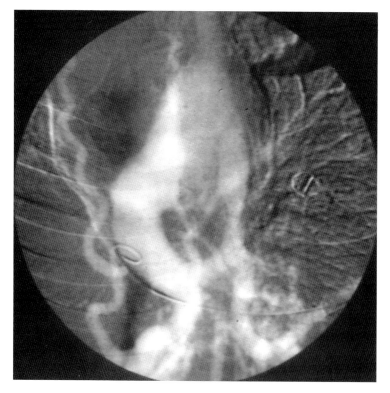

Figure 41 Digital subtraction angiogram of a 14-year-old girl with hypertension and diminished femoral pulses. There is coarction immediately distal to the left subclavian artery. A greatly enlarged internal mammary artery (on the left) provides collateral flow

The condition is relatively common in women who have XO gonadal dysgenesis or Turner's syndrome.

In aortic coarctation, high blood pressure is most marked in the vessels of the upper body proximal to the lesion, the site of which is most often at or just beyond the insertion of the ligamentum arteriosum. A mid-systolic murmur may be audible over the upper anterior chest and back, and aortic systolic murmurs frequently arise from a concurrent bicuspid aortic valve. Enlarged intercostal collateral vessels may be palpable around the chest and there may be overlying vascular bruits.

Pressure levels are much lower in the legs and may be determined with a thigh cuff. Coarctation is usually suspected when the femoral and other leg pulses are either absent, much reduced or delayed compared with pulses in the arm. MRI and spiral CT angiography have proved to be useful techniques for diagnosis, supplementing conventional contrast angiography.

Aortic coarctation is usually detected in the first years of life. Delayed surgical correction of the coarctation leads to residual hypertension in at least 30–50% of patients, who may then require lifelong drug treatment.

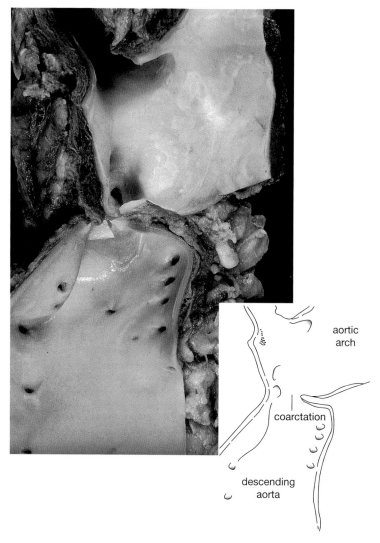

Figure 42 Postmortem thoracic aorta showing a tight coarctation just above the origin of the intercostal arteries. Note the presence of early atheroma above, but not below, the coarctation. The 20-year-old patient died due to aortic dissection; marked left ventricular failure was also present

Interaction with lipids

Patients with raised blood pressure often have other risk factors for atherosclerotic disease. Epidemiological studies have shown a tendency for these factors to cluster so that high blood pressure is associated with high plasma levels of cholesterol, obesity and abnormal glucose tolerance. Interventional trials with antihypertensive drugs alone have shown that the risk of coronary events is reduced, at best, by only one-third to one-half of that expected. There may be benefit in combining antihypertensive treatment with lipid-lowering drugs, and the preliminary evidence from one trial suggests support for this approach.

Cigarette smoking remains the major and most easily altered risk factor for coronary artery disease. It has been estimated that around 30% of all coronary deaths are probably caused by smoking. Population surveys have tended to show that smoking is either unrelated or inversely related to blood pressures. In trials of mild hypertension carried out by the Medical Research Council in the UK, the coronary event rate in male smokers was around twice the rate in non-smokers regardless of treatment, and the difference was emphasized in women. In general, outcome trials have shown that the difference between event rates in smokers with mild hypertension compared with non-smokers is greater than the difference in event rates between active antihypertensive treatment and placebo. Despite the absence of any correlation between smoking and blood pressure in population studies, an association between cigarette smoking and malignant hypertension may be due to atherosclerotic renovascular disease.

Many prospective studies, including the Framingham study, carried out in the developed countries have shown that the risk of cardiovascular disease for a middle-aged man over a period of approximately 10 years shows a ten-fold gradient between those in the lowest quintile of distribution of plasma cholesterol and those in the highest quintile.

Across populations, the major difference in mortality rate due to ischemic heart disease in the Far East compared with Europe and North America appears to be related to differences in average cholesterol levels, as hypertension and cigarette smoking are relatively common in both populations. In Japan, there is an inverse and unexplained relationship between plasma levels of cholesterol and risk of cerebral hemorrhage. Compared with total cholesterol levels, the LDL subfraction is a better predictor of the presence of disease, and prediction is further refined if the ratio of LDL to high-density lipoprotein cholesterol is used. The role of high triglyceride levels as an independent risk factor is still under debate, but is becoming more widely accepted.

The measurement and treatment of raised levels of total and LDL cholesterol with diet and drugs are central to the multiple risk factor approach that is increasingly being used to treat patients who have high blood pressure. Much effort has gone into defining the population subgroups that are at high coronary risk and who merit concurrent treatment with 3-hydroxy-3-methylglutaryl-CoA (HMG-CoA) reductase inhibitors (statins).

Bibliography

Alderman MH. Blood pressure management: individualized treatment based on absolute risk and the potential for benefit. *Ann Intern Med* 1993;119:329–35

Anderson KM, Wilson PWF, Odell PW, Kannel WB. An updated coronary risk profile. A statement for health professionals. *Circulation* 1991;83:356–62

Bamford J, Sandercock P, Dennis M, *et al.* Classification and natural history of clinically identifiable subtypes of cerebral infarction. *Lancet* 1991;337:1521–6

Blaufox MD, Middleton MM, Fine EG. In Laragh JH, Brenner BM, eds. *Hypertension: Pathophysiology, Diagnosis and Management*, 2nd edn. New York: Raven Press, 1996:2005–36

Biglieri EG, Kater CE, Mantero F. Adrenocortical forms of human hypertension. In Laragh JH, Brenner BM, eds. *Hypertension: Pathophysiology, Diagnosis and Management*, 2nd edn. New York: Raven Press, 1996:2145–61

Blood Pressure Lowering Treatment Trialists' Collaboration. Effects of ACE inhibitors, calcium antagonists, and other blood-pressure-lowering drugs: results of prospectively designed overviews of randomised trials. *Lancet* 2000;355:1955–64

Bogousslavsky J, Caplan L, eds. *Stroke Syndromes*. Cambridge: Cambridge University Press, 1995

Bohlen L, De Courten M, Weidmann P. Comparative study of the effect of ACE inhibitors and other antihypertensives on proteinuria in diabetic patients. *Am J Hypertens* 1994;7(Suppl 11):84S–92

Bonelli FS, McKusick MA, Textor SC, *et al.* Renal angioplasty technical results and clinical outcome in 320 patients. *Mayo Clin Proc* 1995;70:1041–52

Boudewijn G, Vasbinder C, Nelemans PJ, *et al.* Diagnostic tests for renal artery stenosis in patients suspected of having renovascular hypertension: a meta-analysis. *Ann Intern Med* 2001;135:401–11

Breyer JA. Medical management of nephropathy in type I diabetes mellitus: current recommendations. *J Am Soc Nephrol* 1995;6:1523–9

Brown MJ, Palmer CR, Castaigne A, *et al.* Morbidity and mortality in patients randomised to double-blind treatment with a long-acting calcium-channel blocker or diuretic in the International Nifedipine GITS study: Intervention as a Goal in Hypertension Treatment (INSIGHT). *Lancet* 2000;356:366–72

Collins R, Peto R, MacMahon S, *et al.* Blood pressure and coronary heart disease. II. *Lancet* 1990;335:827–38

D'Amico G, Minetti L, Ponticelli C, *et al.* Prognostic indicators in idiopathic IgA mesangial nephropathy. *Q J Med* 1986;59:363–78

Dahlöf B, Devereux RB, Kjeldsen SE, the LIFE study group. Cardiovascular morbidity and mortality in the Losartan Intervention For Endpoint reduction in hypertension study (LIFE): a randomised trial against atenolol. *Lancet* 2002;359:995–1003

Dominiczak AF, Lyall F, Morton JJ, *et al.* Blood pressure, left ventricular mass and intracellular calcium in primary hyperparathyroidism. *Clin Sci* 1990;78:127–32

Fisher CM. Lacunar infarcts: a review. *Cerebrovasc Dis* 1991;1:11–20

Haffner SM, Ferrannini E, Hazudu HP, Stern MP. Clustering of cardiovascular risk factors in confirmed prehypertensive individuals. *Hypertension* 1992;20:38–45

Hammond IW, Devereux RB, Alderman MH, et al. The prevalence and correlates of echocardiographic left ventricular hypertrophy among employed patients with uncomplicated hypertension. J Am Coll Cardiol 1986;7:639–50

Hansson L, Zanchetti A, Carruthers SG, et al. Effects of intensive blood pressure lowering and low dose aspirin in patients with hypertension in the Hypertension Optimal Treatment (HOT) randomized trial. Lancet 1998;351:1755–62

Heart Outcomes Prevention Evaluation (HOPE) Study Investigators. Effects of ramipril on cardiovascular and microvascular outcomes in people with diabetes mellitus: results of the HOPE study and MICRO-HOPE substudy. Lancet 2000;355:253–9

Hougen TJ, Sell JE. Recent advances in the diagnosis and treatment of coarctation of the aorta. Curr Opin Cardiol 1995;10:524–9

Humphrey LL, Chan BKS, Sox HC. Postmenopausal hormone replacement therapy and the primary prevention of cardiovascular disease. Ann Intern Med 2002;137: 273–84

Janssen WMT, de Jong PE, de Zeeuw D. Hypertension and renal disease: role of microalbuminuria. J Hypertens 1996;14(Suppl 5):S173–7

Kaplan NM. Management of hypertension in patients with type-2 diabetes mellitus: guidelines based on current evidence. Ann Intern Med 2001;135:1079–83

Kase CS, Caplan LR, eds. Intracerebral Hemorrhage. Boston: Butterworth–Heinemann, 1994

Laragh JH, Brenner BM, eds. Hypertension, vols I & II, 2nd edn. New York: Raven Press, 1995

MacMahon S, Peto R, Cutler J, et al. Blood pressure, stroke and coronary heart disease. I. Lancet 1990;335:765–74

Manger WM, Gifford RW. Pheochromocytoma: a clinical overview. Adrenocortical forms of human hypertension. In Laragh JH, Brenner BM, eds. *Hypertension: Pathophysiology, Diagnosis and Management*, 2nd edn. New York: Raven Press, 1996:2225–44

McGregor E, Isles CG, Lever AF, Murray GD. Retinal changes in malignant hypertension. *Br Med J* 1986;292:233–4

McLenachan JM, Henderson E, Morris KL, Dargie HJ. Ventricular arrhythmias in patients with hypertensive LVH. *N Engl J Med* 1987;317:787–92

Missouris CG, Forbat SM, Singer DRJ, *et al.* Echocardiography over-estimates left ventricular mass: a comparative study with magnetic resonance imaging in patients with hypertension. *J Hypertens* 1996;4:1005–10

MRC/BHF Heart Protection Study of cholesterol lowering with simvastatin in 20 536 high-risk individuals: a randomized placebo-controlled trial. *Lancet* 2002;360:7–22

Mulvany MJ. Resistance vessel structure in hypertension, growth or remodeling. *J Cardiovasc Pharmacol* 1993;22(Suppl 5):S44–7

Nichols AB, Sciacca RR, Weiss MB, *et al.* Effect of left ventricular hypertrophy on myocardial blood flow and ventricular performance in systemic hypertension. *Circulation* 1980;62:329–40

O'Rourke MF, Kelly RP. Wave reflection in the systemic circulation, and its implication in ventricular function in man. *J Hypertens* 1993;11:327–37

Pahor M, Psaty BM, Alderman MH, *et al.* Health outcomes associated with calcium antagonists compared with other first-line antihypertensive therapies: a meta-analysis of randomised controlled trials. *Lancet* 2000;356:1949–54

Parati G, Omboni S, Mancia G. Difference between office and ambulatory blood pressure and response to antihypertensive treatment. *J Hypertens* 1996;14:791–7

Petrie JC, O'Brien ET, Littler WA, de Swiet M, for the British Hypertension Society. Recommendations on blood pressure measurement. *Br Med J* 1986;293:611–15

Peart S, Brennan PJ, Broughton P, *et al.* Medical Research Council trial of treatment in older adults: principal results. *Br Med J* 1992;304:505–12

Pederson TR. Primary prevention of cardiovascular disease. *J Hypertens* 1996;14(Suppl 5):S195–200

Pickering TG. Which measures of blood pressure give the best prediction of target organ damage and prognosis? In Pickering TG, ed. *Ambulatory Monitoring and Blood Pressure Variability*. London: Science Press, 1991:13.1–15

Prospective Studies Collaboration. Age-specific relevance of usual blood pressure to vascular mortality: a meta-analysis of individual data for one million adults in 61 prospective studies. *Lancet* 2002;360:1903–13

Reichard P, Nilsson B-Y, Rosenquist U. The effect of long-term intensified treatment in the development of microvascular complications of diabetes mellitus. *N Engl J Med* 1993;329:304–9

Rossouw JE, Anderson GL, *et al.* Risks and benefits of estrogen plus progestin in healthy postmenopausal women: principal results from the Women's Health Initiative Randomized Controlled Trial. *J Am Med Assoc* 2002;288:321–33

Sacks FM, Pfeffer MA, Moye LA, *et al.* The effect of pravastatin on coronary events after myocardial infarction in patients with average cholesterol levels. *N Engl J Med* 1996;335:1001–9

Scandinavian Simvastatin Survival Study (4S). Randomized trial of cholesterol-lowering in 4444 patients with coronary heart disease. *Lancet* 1994;344:1383–9

Semple PF. Mineralocorticoid excess. In James VHT, ed. *The Adrenal Gland*, 2nd edn. New York: Raven Press, 1992:373–89

Semple PF, Dominiczak AF. Detection and treatment of renovascular disease: 40 years on. *J Hypertens* 1994;12:729–34

Shepherd J, Cobbe SM, Ford I, *et al*. Prevention of coronary heart disease with pravastatin in men with hypercholesterolemia. *N Engl J Med* 1995;333:1301–7

Skinhoj E, Strandgaard S. Pathogenesis of hypertensive encephalopathy. *Lancet* 1973;I:461–2

Smith MC, Dunn MJ. Hypertension in renal parenchymal disease. In Laragh JH, Brenner BM, eds. *Hypertension: Pathophysiology, Diagnosis and Management*, 2nd edn. New York: Raven Press, 1996:2081–102

Steward PM. Cortisol as a mineralocorticoid in human disease. *J Steroid Biochem Mol Biol* 1999;69:403–8

Swales J, ed. *Textbook of Hypertension*. London: Blackwell Scientific Publishers, 1994

Staessen JA, Gasowski J, Wang JG, *et al*. Risks of untreated and treated isolated systolic hypertension in the elderly: meta-analysis of outcome trials. *Lancet* 2000;355:865–72

Systolic Hypertension in the Elderly Program (SHEP). Prevention of stroke by antihypertensive drug treatments: final results from the Systolic Hypertension in the Elderly Program (SHEP). *J Am Med Assoc* 1991;265:3255–64

Tegtmeyer CJ, Matsumoto AH, Angle JF. Percutaneous transluminal angioplasty in fibrous dysplasia. In Novick AC, ed. *Renal Vascular Disease*. London: WB Saunders, 1996:363–83

The ALLHAT Officers and Coordinators for the ALLHAT Collaborative Research Group. Major cardiovascular events in hypertensive patients randomized to doxazosin vs chlorthalidone. The Antihypertensive and Lipid-Lowering Treatment to Prevent Heart Attack Trial (ALLHAT). *J Am Med Assoc* 2000;283:1967–75

The Diabetes Control and Complications Trial Research Group. The effect of intensive treatment of diabetes on the development and progression of long-term complications in insulin-dependent diabetes mellitus. *N Engl J Med* 1993;329:977–86

US Preventative Task Force. Postmenopausal hormone replacement therapy for primary prevention of chronic conditions: recommendations and rationale. *Ann Intern Med* 2002;137:834–9

Van Jaarsveld BC, Krijnen P, Pieterman H, *et al.* The effect of balloon angioplasty on hypertension atherosclerotic renal artery stenosis. *N Engl J Med* 2000;342:1007–14

Whitworth JA. Mechanisms of glucocorticoid-induced hypertension. *Kidney Int* 1987;31:1213–24

Wolf PA, d'Agostino RB, Belanger AJ, Kannel WB. Probability of stroke: a risk profile from the Framingham Study. *Stroke* 1991;22:312–18

Index